W9-BQX-946

OVEREXTENDED AND UNDERNOURISHED

A Self-Care Guide for People in Helping Roles

Dennis Portnoy, MFCC

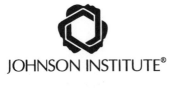

JOHNSON INSTITUTE®

Minneapolis

Copyright © 1996 by Johnson Insitute-QVS, Inc. All rights reserved world-wide. No part of this manuscript may be reproduced or transmitted in any form or by any means, electronic or mechanical, including photocopying or recording, by and information storage and retrieval system, without express permission from the publisher.

Johnson Institute-QVS, Inc.
7205 Ohms Lane
Minneapolis, MN 55439-2159
(800) 231-5165 or (612) 831-1630

Library of Congress Cataloging-in-Publication Data
Portnoy, Dennis, 1951–
    Overextended and Undernourished : a self-care guide for people in
helping roles / Dennis Portnoy
        p. cm.
    ISBN 1-56246-115-X
    1. Human services personnel--Job Stress--United States. 2. Human ser-vices personnel--United States--Psychology. 3. Caregivers--United States--Psychology. 4. Stress management--United States. 5. Self-help techniques--United States. 6. Burn out (Psychology)--Prevention.
    I. Title
    HV40.8.U6P67 1996
    361.3'019--dc20
    95-53695
                                                                                                    CIP

Cover and page design: Crombie Design

Printed in the United States of America

For Anna

Contents

INTRODUCTION
Please Read This First

This book is designed to guide people in helping roles as they deal with a unique set of problems they may encounter—problems that arise from within, rather than from an external caregiving situation itself. Oftentimes, difficulties originating from internal and external sources are interwoven, increasing the negative effects of stress and leading to burnout.

I wrote this book for those who help others on a personal or professional basis. I have used the terms "those in helping roles" to cover three groups of helpers, or caregivers, who may find the information in this book particularly useful. Basically, I wrote the book for helping professionals: counselors, medical and nursing personnel, rescue workers, physical and occupational therapists, teachers, social workers, all those who are involved in the work of helping people. Others who may find this book useful include persons who are helping friends or family members. There are also people who, in effect, are natural healers. While these individuals are not necessarily helping professionals or caregivers, they have a comforting presence. These "natural healers" are also externally directed, and focused on the needs of others. Therefore, they encounter the challenges unique to helping roles.

In addition to the challenges inherent in helping others, many people in helping roles also deal with the added stress of carrying out their roles in dysfunctional settings. In her book, *Home Away From Home*, Janet Woititz describes addictive organizations, for example, as having a crisis orientation, rigid rules, poor communication among departments, employing dysfunctional behaviors such as perfectionism, and continuously doing more than is expected.

Some people in helping roles work with those who suffer from intense physical and emotional trauma. Helpers working in these intense situations may experience flashbacks and become numb themselves—symptoms associated with secondary stress and compassion fatigue.

People in helping roles tend to have a high burnout rate. In the early stages of burnout, life may seem less enjoyable to the helper and he or she begins to feel agitated and tired. In later stages of burnout, however, the helper actually may become ill more frequently, feel overwhelmed, have strained relationships, decreased productivity, and/or sudden outbursts of anger.

Help is generally available, but even the best stress-reduction techniques have limited impact for a helper unless he or she resolves a crucial issue: *the self-imposed stress underlying the burnout.* Over ten years of counseling people in helping roles and conducting training for them have taught me the importance of addressing the self-imposed stress that creates difficulties for so many caregivers.

Some of the personality characteristics that contribute to burnout are: denial; need to control; difficulty in delegating work to others; poor boundary affirmation; ongoing and intense self-criticism; lack of leisure-time interests and pursuits; inability to develop nourishing friendships and intimate relationships; and over-identification with the role of giver.

My intention in this book is not to generalize about complex dynamics or reduce them to quick fixes or formulas, but to identify some behavior patterns, personal histories, and helping situations that I believe are worthy of consideration by anyone in a helping role.

This book is divided into four chapters that address the unique challenges encountered by people in helping roles. My hope is that the information provided here will guide people in helping roles as they learn to recognize and better understand the beliefs, attitudes, and behaviors that increase the negative effects of stress. I also hope that this book will provide a source of guidance to helpers as they look at concrete ways they can improve their abilities to set limits, resolve conflicts, manage objectives, and take care of their own needs for support, care, self-esteem, and comfort.

I. Destructive Habits and Self-Imposed Stress

This chapter describes personality traits and habits that undermine effectiveness, create harmful stress, and lead to burnout. It identifies the tendency of some people to take on too much responsibility and/or rely on control; and it distinguishes between healthy and unhealthy giving. Two dysfunctional helping styles—people-pleasing and absorbing—are identified, along with problems related to each style and the healing tasks that help to counteract them.

II. Accepting and Revealing Vulnerability

This section outlines the process of identifying and counteracting attitudes that lead to over-identification with a helper role. Using examples from his counseling practice,

3

the author provides specific help for learning how to counteract excessive reliance on "being strong" and "in control."

III. Recreating the Familiar: Childhood Scenarios at Work

This chapter reveals how the roles people play as adults may evolve from the roles assigned by families during childhood. It identifies specific roles that relate to unhealthy helping: the good child, the responsible child, the healer, the peacekeeper.

IV. Saying "Yes" to Yourself

Chapter IV provides special tools for caregivers to enable them to take good care of themselves as they care for others. Topics addressed include: distinguishing between enlightened self-interest and selfishness; setting limits; building stress-resilience; identifying emotional needs; and getting needs met.

CHAPTER I

Destructive Habits and Self-Imposed Stress

Exaggerated Responsibility

Jim, a 33-year-old clergyman, came to me for counseling because of sleep difficulties and stress. At the time, Jim was working 12-hour days and was taking on a multitude of tasks unrelated to his role as pastor of a large suburban church. He was even spending several hours of his time each week answering routine phone calls in the church office.

Looking tired and anxious, Jim explained to me that essentially he was dedicating his entire life to his work because the church he served was having severe financial problems and on the verge of collapse due to mismanagement by the board. Although Jim acknowledged that he was not the cause of the financial or management problems challenging the church community, he clearly felt that it was his job to save the church. As we talked further about his situation and his feelings, Jim revealed to me that if the problems of the church were not solved at once, he would regard himself as a complete failure.

Jim is reliable, sensitive, and devoted to his parishioners. Many of his personal traits are, in fact, very useful in his role as a clergyman. Unmoderated or used improperly, however, these personal traits can become destructive to him and to those who depend on him as well.

The tendency to take on too much responsibility creates stress in both personal and professional relationships.

When someone else is having a bad day, the overly responsible person may actually feel an obligation to have a bad day as well. People who take on too much responsibility for the feelings of others might, for example, feel that it is their "duty" to put others at ease, protect them from the realities of accountability and criticism, and offer too much help to them in carrying out their tasks and responsibilities.

People who have an exaggerated sense of responsibility also tend to have a high level of concern with "being strong" for others. They may feel that it is extremely important to always be perceived by others as "having it all together" and to know that others rely on them for advice. For this reason, they work hard to avoid displaying any kind of weakness.

People who feel unrealistically responsible for the feelings of others may be motivated by guilt, duty, obligation, or fear. Indeed, when a person with an exaggerated sense of responsibility is unable to "fix" another person's problems, he or she tends to feel at fault for the entire situation.

Over-Reliance on Control

A common characteristic of people who take on too much responsibility is their over-reliance on control, primarily to ward off feelings of powerlessness and/or to establish a sense of order. Controllers are likely to perceive themselves as indispensable and tend to feel that they must do everything themselves. They have difficulty delegating and asking for help and they truly believe that tasks will be carried out correctly only if they are doing the tasks themselves or are in a position to control those who are charged with the tasks. Controllers also find uncertainty very difficult, if not intolerable, and tend to get into power struggles related to this controlling behavior.

It's not surprising that stress management techniques are only minimally effective with people who do not address their inability to relinquish control. These people simply cannot relax enough to benefit from stress management until they feel safe—in other words, until they know that it's okay to let go of control.

Rescuing Behavior

Jim, the clergyman, was a rescuer. For many people, like Jim, who cross the line from healthy to unhealthy helping, rescuing behavior represents a way to push feelings of helplessness out of awareness.

When rescuing behavior leads to order in the midst of real danger, uncertainty, change, or chaos, it can be functional. But when the dangers that represent a perceived need for rescue are exaggerated, the rescuing behavior that results is likely to be self-defeating.

In Jim's case, the appropriate helping behavior would have been directed only toward the personal problems of his parishioners, not to the financial problems of the church. Business affairs related to the functioning of the church were, by definition and through job description, the responsibility of the governing board of the church. Given the situation, the most useful task Jim could perform was really quite clear: convene a group of responsible parishioners to take over the task of electing a new board or demand better management from the current board.

Jim expected disaster when he surrendered a degree of control to the church board. In fact, the business affairs of the church could be put in order by the board with relative ease. Once Jim was able to let go, and let others in the church community use their resources to restore order to the finances of the church, he began to relax and pay attention to his own needs. This new sense of priority and balance in Jim's life helped him take care of his own needs and fulfill his primary responsibility to his parishioners.

Breaking Free of Exaggerated Responsibility

People who have a tendency to take on too much responsibility usually find it helpful to identify and challenge family expectations—particularly expectations that develop when one takes on an adult responsibility while still a child.

In Jim's case, he got the important start he needed toward making positive changes in his life when he carefully considered the connection between his adult behavior and his upbringing. Jim grew up feeling responsible for the problems in his family. At the age of eleven, he experienced the trauma of having his retarded brother removed from the family home and sent to a residential facility in another town. A year after that event, Jim's parents divorced. During this time of change, Jim's parents apparently failed to reassure him or consider how these family crises were affecting their young son. Not wanting to further burden his parents, Jim stuffed his feelings related to each of these two major life events.

The traumatic events in Jim's childhood ultimately resulted in his feeling helpless, out of control, and responsible for the family's problems. Like many children, Jim felt it was his "duty" to make things better for his family. Furthermore, he felt like a failure for not being able to keep the family together.

Jim's extreme rescuing behavior as an adult in a helping role was a subconscious way to exercise control and avoid feelings of helplessness in situations that felt chaotic or uncertain to him. Much of the work in counseling focused on Jim identifying how his current behavior was linked to specific events in his upbringing, and how he was—in ways he carried out in his work responsibilities—recreating familiar themes from his past. I frequently pointed out to Jim the ways in which he apparently felt obligated to others. He began to understand how "feeling obligated" had become a familiar—and therefore comfortable— feeling for him.

As we focused on Jim's feelings about recognizing and challenging his beliefs, he realized that he felt like a failure by not "saving" the church himself. He also came to see how, on an emotional level, the potential collapse of the church he was serving triggered feelings he associated with the collapse of his family twenty years earlier.

During therapy, I engaged Jim in a role play exercise, asking him to imagine saying the following to his parents: "I love you, but it is not my responsibility to make things all right for you." Initially, Jim felt guilty for even uttering the words. I then posed the following question to him: "Jim, what do you think may have happened to you as a youngster if you had been less responsible?" Jim replied: "I would have felt that I had failed my family."

Over time, Jim began to realize that his worth as a person was not totally dependent on his "being responsible for others." He also recognized how, for him, an exaggerated sense of responsibility protected him from being overwhelmed by feelings of helplessness. Gaining access to feelings of helplessness often helps people identify the beliefs and fears that underlie the exaggerated responsibility habit. Jim was able to grasp that the problems in his family were not his fault. He realized that he was not responsible for his family's problems and was not, contrary to his long-held belief, a failure.

A Note about Healthy and Unhealthy Giving

Mary, a 41-year-old social worker was learning the difference between healthy and unhealthy giving "on the job." Her client, a 43-year-old woman with muscular dystrophy, was distressed at having been refused car insurance. Mary's immediate impulse was to make everything okay and to neatly "fix" her client's dilemma by making several phone calls for her. But Mary realized that her response was beyond the scope of healthy helping. Instead of rushing in to "fix" the situation for her client, Mary recommended to her that she contact her own attorney for assistance in handling the situation.

Like Mary, many people in helping roles may confuse healthy and unhealthy giving. This confusion leads to burnout for the helper and has the effect of inhibiting those who are receiving help from appropriately taking responsibility for themselves.

Unhealthy giving by those in helping roles is characterized by the following:

- Excessive need to be needed—in other words, feeling worthwhile only if needed by others.

- Doing too much for another person in the process of helping him or her, thus preventing that person from taking responsibility and fully achieving all that is possible.

- Focusing on the needs and reactions of others to the extent of losing sight of one's own needs, perceptions, limitations, and feelings.

On the other hand, healthy giving by those in helping roles is characterized by the following:

- Supporting another person to be the best that he or she can be.

- Recognizing and valuing one's own needs, perceptions, limitations, and feelings.

- Self-compassion.

- Ability and willingness (of the helper) to ask for help.

People Pleasing: Addiction to Harmony

Being aware of other people's needs is generally a positive attribute, particularly when carrying out a helping role. But when a person's awareness of the needs of others consistently takes precedence over his or her own needs, it can lead to self-neglect and can prevent the person receiving help from taking responsibility for himself or herself. Focusing too much on pleasing others can undermine the helper's ability to set limits and, consequently, can lead to burnout.

People pleasing includes keeping the focus on others by being attentive, accommodating, agreeable, and compliant, even when to do so is to compromise one's own priorities, goals, and tasks. Excessive focus on others may be a way of getting approval and love and avoiding difficult emotions.

Dawn, a 43-year-old manager had difficulty saying "no" to anyone, which caused problems for her in both professional and personal relationships. When Dawn's company promoted her and transferred her to another city, she did not realize that she would be facing an unrealistic work load in her new job. Several key employees had left the company a month before she arrived, creating a number of unfinished projects and a staggering work load for Dawn.

Dawn prided herself on her record as a good, productive worker. She had very high expectations for her own performance and was extremely self-critical. But the growing work load in her new job was so overwhelming to her that she began filing portions of work away, fully intending to get to it eventually. As the file of incomplete work grew and Dawn became more and more overwhelmed with her job, she continued to act as if everything was fine. She felt that to do otherwise or even suggest to others that she was frustrated would make her appear weak or incompetent. Dawn wanted her new colleagues to like and respect her. Simply stated, Dawn was overly concerned about other people's perceptions of her. She was convinced that asking for help and/or saying "no" to a coworker's request would result in people thinking she was weak.

Janet, a 55-year-old supervisor for a utility company, grew up with parents who frequently argued with each other and attempted to get her to choose sides. Consequently, Janet coped by never making waves and by carefully monitoring the responses of everyone around her. Janet's attempts to have harmony at all costs interfered with many aspects of her life, including her ability to delegate authority—a critical and very necessary task in her work.

When ongoing conflict developed between two employees in Janet's department, it was her job to enforce existing company policy and help others resolve their differences within those parameters. But because Janet felt anxious around confrontation, she did not handle her supervisory role effectively. Instead of facilitating a productive resolution between the two employees that would benefit the work situation and the company, Janet focused on trying to get the two employees to ignore their conflict, forget about their anger with each other, and become trusting friends.

Many people pleasers allow others to mistreat them in their efforts to keep things on an even keel. They smooth things over and avoid "making waves" in order to avoid confrontation. Like having radar, they are extremely alert— or hypervigilant—to the moods and feelings of other people. People who are hypervigilant constantly monitor their own thoughts, speech, and actions, carefully watching for the reactions of others. Because their actions are so often based on how others perceive them, people pleasers are not really in charge of their own lives.

Some people develop the habit of hypervigilance out of fear of separation. June, a 36-year-old therapist, grew up feeling like an outsider with her family and her peers. The slightest tension or separation made her feel that she would be excluded and abandoned. Consequently, June always focused her energies on putting people at ease. The difficulty she had tolerating any break in contact from others continued into her adulthood. In counseling, June explored her fears and beliefs, as well as her need for approval. Becoming more aware of her hypervigilance and working with "The Scanner Exercise" in this section of the book, helped June learn to be "at odds" with others. She also learned to appreciate her own differences, even those differences that others may criticize or dislike.

The Healing Task: Tolerating Discord and Saying "No"

In order to bring about positive change for themselves and the people they help, those who have developed the people-pleasing habit must learn to tolerate discord and they also must learn to say "no." People fall into rescuing and the pleasing habit because they cannot tolerate tension, uncertainty, confrontation, and/or separation. The attributes that helped Dawn, the manager, get promoted in her job also created problems for her on the job and in her life. She relied on rescuing and people pleasing in order to relieve tension and/or avoid conflicts she feared would lead to separation from others. Dawn needed to identify and counteract the outdated beliefs that fueled her fears.

In therapy, Dawn explored her childhood role as the "good child," and the parental messages that had the effect of stifling her assertiveness. Dawn focused on the expectations of her parents and how her self-esteem was based on the judgments of others. Her parents had continually stressed to her that it is wrong to disappoint others. She discovered that her parents and other authority figures in her life had placed unrealistic expectations on her.

It was necessary for Dawn to allow herself to experience resentment for having grown up with parents who had unfair expectations of her. Throughout her childhood, Dawn felt guilty when those around her were upset because she was expected to always "be good" and never disappoint people. She came to realize that the only times in her childhood that she received attention or felt special were those times when her parents judged her to be a "good girl."

Many people pleasers need to learn how to accept and appreciate the full range of their experience and emotions. Dawn grew up suppressing anger, irritability, and aggressive feelings. In our counseling sessions, Dawn learned—perhaps for the first time in her life—that it is okay to disagree with others. Accepting this helped her begin to accept herself in situations when she made mistakes. I encouraged her to actually practice being less agreeable in her normal interactions with others and to pay attention to the feelings that arise. When I challenged her belief that saying "no" means hurting others, Dawn discovered that underlying her concern about hurting people was a fear that they would reject her.

I asked Dawn to imagine saying "no" to a coworker who requested her help and to practice saying this: "I'm busy right now and unable to help you; could you ask someone else?" This exercise led her to realize how deeply entrenched in her life were her family's messages that she should never disappoint others.

In our counseling sessions, I asked Janet, the supervisor, what she thought might have happened in her family had she "rocked the boat" as a child. I asked her the following question: "Janet, what would have happened to you as a child if you had disagreed with your parents or otherwise expressed an opposing view?" Recalling her childhood evoked in Janet fears about lack of order (discord) and about situations getting totally out of control. Janet realized that she did not feel emotionally safe as a child, and that discord evoked feelings of powerlessness in her.

By recognizing the "peacekeeper" role she played in her early years and by separating her past from her present day reality, Janet learned to better tolerate inevitable tense moments in the workplace and to put far less emphasis on being a people pleaser. She saw how being hypervigilant was related to her inability to tolerate any level of tension whatsoever. Subconsciously, Janet believed that "making waves" and "being at odds" with others would result in painful consequences for her. In our counseling sessions, Janet practiced, through role play, confronting and disagreeing with people, which enabled her to recognize that her fears were based on outdated childhood perceptions.

Exercise 1: The Scanner

In order to avoid feelings of tension, minimize anxiety, and/or insure emotional safety, people who are hypervigilant continually adapt their responses to what they think others want to hear. Consequently, they may say "yes" when they mean "no." When hypervigilance is familiar behavior, it may not seem at all excessive or inappropriate to the person who practices it.

How often and to what degree do you scan your responses and the responses of others?

_____

_____

When you are being hypervigilant, what sensations and emotions do you notice in yourself? For example, are your eyes more alert and watching others?

_____

_____

What situations cause you to be hypervigilant?

_____

_____

Imagine being in these situations and not being hypervigilant. How does this make you feel?

_____

_____

Exercise 2: Saying "No"

Can you think of situations when you felt like saying "no" but stopped yourself?

Now, practice expressing an opinion that is different from the opinion of someone else as if that person is with you in this moment. (In practicing, think of expressing yourself to a person you do not know particularly well.)

As you express your opinion to this person, what are you feeling?

_____

_____

Imagine facing that person and saying to him or her: "It is okay for me to disagree with you."

_____

_____

What is your worst fear of how this person may respond to you?

_____

_____

Do your thoughts and feelings remind you of any experience with significant people in your past?

_____

_____

Absorbing Other People's Feelings and Problems

Frank is a 48-year-old social worker for a county hospital. His job is particulary demanding, for it combines the daily care of hospitalized patients as well as the followup care of patients after they leave the hospital. Frank continually interacts with doctors, nurses, family members, and community agencies. Due to budget cuts, he and two other social workers carry a work load that formerly required the services of five professional social workers.

Frank's workplace is stressful in itself, but his temperament makes his job even more difficult. Frank has difficulty setting limits; he brings work problems home and is unable to maintain an appropriate distance from his patients, both during and after the workday.

Frank absorbs the problems and challenges of his patients to the extent that he becomes physically and emotionally drained. In fact, he often feels personally responsible for the discomfort of his patients. For example, when a patient confides his or her feelings of sadness to Frank, he becomes sad himself, taking on the full impact of that individual's pain.

Absorbers often feel emotionally drained because they are over-involved with others. One nurse, for example, complained in therapy about waking up several nights a week to a feeling that her patients were right there in her bedroom, needing attention and care.

Like many people who absorb the problems of others, Frank becomes so focused on other people that he forgets his own preferences, goals, and desires. At times Frank adopts other people's attitudes, values, and emotions—to the degree that he is unable to distinguish between the feelings and thoughts of others and feelings and thoughts of his own.

Strengthening Boundaries and Establishing Autonomy

Absorbers characteristically have difficulty defining their boundaries. When boundaries are clear, people have "protective filters" that enable them to set limits and to be compassionate and open to others without losing their separate identities. But when boundaries are unclear, people may do some or all of the following: reveal personal information to casual acquaintances, allow others to control their lives, let themselves be consumed by another person, fail to recognize intrusive behavior, and/or fail to stand up for themselves.

Frank continually gave to others, not even recognizing his need for distance. He completely lost touch with his own perceptions, needs, and limitations, particularly when helping people in pain. Boundary and autonomy issues are often linked to upbringing. Frank grew up being a confidante to his mother. In confiding her problems to Frank, his mother crossed a significant parent-child boundary, elevating Frank to the level of peer. Her over-involvement with him was intrusive and interfered with the establishment of clear boundaries. Frank was so attuned to his mother's needs that he experienced her problems as if they were his own.

Taking on other people's problems and putting his own needs on hold was a thoroughly familiar role for Frank. In adulthood, he recreated his family role in his adult relationships. Consequently, his relationships were onesided and unsatisfying. He was drawn to people who were needy, self-centered, and rarely considered his needs.

In our counseling sessions, I focused on strengthening Frank's boundaries and tasks designed to help him separate from his mother. Frank needed to learn that his needs and feelings are as important as those of anyone else. He also needed to learn that his mother's over-involvement weakened his boundaries, preventing him from developing an identity separate from hers.

I pointed out to Frank that his mother's behavior in confiding to him essentially robbed him of a childhood and how, consequently, he came to be valued primarily for his helpfulness. Frank had difficulty recognizing his mother's unfairness because he had never experienced truly nurturing parenting.

I suggested to Frank an exercise that teaches people about the obstacles they put in the way that interfere with the establishment of clear boundaries. I asked Frank to imagine saying this to his mother: "I care about you, but your pain is not my pain." This exercise is not designed to make people insensitive, but to establish a healthy distance that ultimately benefits everyone involved in a helping realtionship.

People who have absorber tendencies have a particularly strong reaction to this exercise. They may feel guilty and responsible for the other person's happiness and they may have difficulty tolerating thoughts of separation. When "absorbers" think about distancing from people who are important in their lives, they tend to become fearful of being rejected or abandoned by these people.

In fact, Frank recoiled when asked to repeat this statement to his mother. He felt guilty for saying no to people who needed him. Further exploration revealed that his reluctance to do the exercise stemmed from his belief that he had no right to resent, or even question, his mother. Eventually, however, Frank was able to make this statement without feeling guilty. In order to counteract an erroneous belief he had about himself and his worth, I suggested that he repeat the following on a daily basis: "My value does not depend on my ability to take care of others."

Frank subsequently began to separate from his mother's pain and pay more attention to his own feelings and needs.

His boundaries became stronger when he realized how his behavior had been influenced by his upbringing. It was important that Frank "experience" the unfairness of his mother's reliance on him, as well as her neglect of his needs. Coming to terms with the resentment and hurt he felt—not simply his conceptual understanding of his past— enabled him to let go of unhealthy helping behavior. Establishing a clear, separate identity and firm boundaries are the keys to counteracting the absorbing habit.

CHAPTER II

Accepting and Revealing Vulnerability

"Being Strong" and "In Control"

The first section of this book describes how an exaggerated sense of responsibility is likely to cause people in helping roles to over-identify with "being strong" and "in control." Some people who are drawn to helping roles actually derive their identity and self-worth from being strong and in control. Furthermore, these people may also associate vulnerable feelings with weakness, dependency, and being out of control. They are likely to suppress the softer, more tender aspects of their personalities in order to reinforce their sense of personal strength. The need to always be strong and in control often creates tension in relationships and causes the kind of stress that leads to burnout.

Some of the characteristics of overly-responsible, strong people are:

- they feel responsible for the happiness (or unhappiness) of others

- they have difficulty accepting their own limitations

- they require others to need them in order to feel worthwhile

- they are often motivated by obligation or guilt.

- they distrust the reliability of others

- they equate needing others with being weak

The ongoing need to be strong and in control can create a sense of order and provide a way to escape or deny the feelings of powerlessness that may be associated with one's upbringing. This often occurs with children who grow up with parents who disapprove of their expressions of sadness, anxiety, or fear. In families already dealing with high levels of stress, fear, or uncertainty, the threat of situations getting "out of control" can be very real and very frightening as well. An example of this would be a child who believes he or she has to be strong, responsible, and/or able to provide all the right answers to insure that his or her parent does not get drunk.

People learn to relinquish the need to control and an over-identification with being strong when they learn to accept their vulnerable emotions. The path to self-healing also involves recognizing and challenging expectations of self as well as beliefs and fears about failing and being weak. Certain childhood fears and memories are triggered in adult life. It follows, then, that conscious efforts to relinquish control may trigger and even heighten existing anxieties regarding loss of control. Most people find it easier to work on this challenging task with a therapist or a close friend because that kind of support feels safe to them.

Mark, a 34-year-old police dispatcher, reluctantly sought counseling because of marital problems. Though he and his wife were having significant problems in their relationship, Mark hadn't wanted to seek counseling, preferring to work things out "at home, without involving other people."

Mark appeared to be "strong" and "in control," as evidenced by his braced body language and the way he kept a tight lid on his emotions. When I asked him to describe his parents and his upbringing, he described a family that strongly emphasized self-sufficiency, but was not open to the expression of feelings. In Mark's family, needing others and asking for help were considered signs of weakness.

As Mark's therapist, my response to him was different from the responses he was accustomed to, in that I acknowledged and accepted his vulnerable feelings. In time, this acceptance helped Mark, himself, accept the softer, more vulnerable aspects of his personality. We explored the expectations his parents communicated to him early in his life and confronted deep-seated beliefs that had shaped his life. Then I gently challenged Mark's belief that needing help from others and making mistakes meant that he was a weak and ineffective person.

In therapy, I did a simple exercise with Mark that helped him discover the hidden assumptions that prevented him from accepting his vulnerability and relinquishing control. I asked him to state the following half sentences aloud, filling in the second part of the sentence with whatever phrase immediately came to his mind—without any concern for making logical sense:

Needing someone means that I am...

If I am not strong, then I am...

Mark completed the sentences in the following ways:

"Needing someone...means that I am weak."

"If I am not strong...then I am a failure."

I then asked Mark the following questions:

What would it be like to rely on someone and talk about sadness or fear?

What is wrong with failing?

What does it feel like not to be able to help someone who asks for your help?

Clearly, Mark was not accustomed to focusing on his own needs or feelings. I asked him to consider how he felt when he thought about these questions. He responded by saying that the questions made him feel guilty, uncomfortable, and disgusted. Mark grew up feeling guilty and that he was a failure if he let someone down who was counting on him.

I then asked Mark what he feared would happen if he relinquished control and became more vulnerable and less self-sufficient. Much to his surprise, he discovered that not being self-sufficient and always in control meant—for him—that no one would "be there" for him and that others could take advantage of him. Underneath Mark's strong, controlled demeanor was a subconscious fear of being helpless and alone.

Mark needed a safe environment in which to experience these emotions and learn some new things as well. Most important, Mark needed to learn that people can be reliable and trustworthy, and that letting go of his reliance on control would not result in the collapse of his world.

Mark also began to realize that the expectations of his parents were unfair and unattainable. Many people have great difficulty admitting that the expectations their parents had of them were inappropriate. At any stage of life, it is difficult to admit that one's parents made mistakes. Mark's feelings of resentment toward his family for always expecting him to be strong actually helped him to make a positive change in his life. Though it was difficult for him to acknowledge resentment of his parents, Mark felt freer when he realized that he was not responsible for family problems.

The familiar feels normal, so people who grow up with perfectionistic standards and a lack of support do not recognize an injustice. As these people move through their lives, they tend to behave in ways that sustain the familiar.

Exercise 3: Expressing Vulnerability

The messages we receive when we are children have a powerful effect on us as we grow older. Regardless of how parents convey negative messages about vulnerability, the impact these messages have on children is significant.

When children are denied the opportunity to acknowledge and/or express their feelings and emotions, they are likely to grow up having great difficulty associated with the following life skills: acknowledging needs, relying on others, and expressing tender emotions and feelings. Some people, for example, grow up learning that it is wrong to display vulnerability. A parent may threaten the whimpering or crying child with a statement like this: "If you're going to sit there and cry, I'll give you something to really cry about."

Allow your mind to drift back to childhood, to a period in your life between the ages of seven and twelve. Imagine yourself during that period of time expressing feelings of sadness and anxiety to your parents, then ask yourself these questions:

How would they respond to you?

_____

_____

How did they respond to their own fears and vulnerable emotions?

_____

_____

How much room did they allow for making mistakes?

_____

_____

Perfectionistic Expectations and Self-Compassion

People who over-identify with "being strong" and "in control" frequently have difficulty accepting their own limitations and are likely to be perfectionistic. It is important to make a distinction between perfection and excellence, yet many people find it difficult to do so. Here's a useful distinction between the two: The pursuit of excellence allows for error and self-compassion; perfectionists, on the other hand, cannot tolerate their own weaknesses. While perfectionists have compassion for others, they have little or no compassion for themselves. Furthermore, perfectionists are often highly self-critical, while attempting to live up to unrealistic standards. Cultivating self-compassion helps a person break free of harsh, perfectionistic expectations and the need to always "be strong."

Lee, a 32-year-old music teacher became ill after pushing herself for years to be "the best." While recuperating, she realized how her perfectionistic expectations had contributed to her illness. "I was trying," said Lee, "to live up to an image of how I should be, rather than accepting my limitations. When I was not living up to my standards, I viewed myself as a total failure. No matter how much I accomplished, a little voice in my head always told me that I was not doing enough."

Sylvia, a 50-year-old supervisor at a health clinic, was given the responsibility for conducting a staff meeting each morning. "I was anxious about this task," said Sylvia, "because I had no previous experience conducting meetings. I spent a week criticizing myself for not having skills I was never taught. I finally realized that I would be very understanding and patient with anyone else facing the same new challenge I was facing."

Exercise 4: Distinguishing Between Realistic and Unrealistic Expectations

Under each of the categories listed below, indicate the expectations that these groups of people had of you when you were a child.

Parents

_____

_____

Teachers

_____

_____

Society

_____

_____

Religious Authorities

_____

_____

When you have completed your lists, consider how the expectations you grew up with reflect the expectations you currently have of yourself.

After completing this exercise, a clergyman wrote the following: "When we were asked to list the expectations others had of us as children, I groaned inside. Under the Parents category, I wrote:

Be perfect—Be responsible—Be the leader.

Under the Teachers category, I wrote:

Be quiet—Do good work—Think well.

Under the Religious Authority Category, I wrote:

Do not screw up—Do not bother us with problems—You are on your own."

The clergyman continued, " As I did this exercise, I could feel anger surfacing and I began to make a list of the expectations I now have from my congregation. I realized that I felt trapped and unable to be authentic. As I looked at the list, I made a connection that I had not made before: the expectations from my parents in the past and my congregation in the present put me at very high risk for burnout. I saw how I translated my old tapes from my parents to my congregation. The expectations to be perfect, responsible, and a leader created overwhelming tensions inside of me. After seeing my lists, I now recognize how unrealistic those demands are."

Core Assumptions

Throughout this book, I emphasize the importance of discovering, then changing, core beliefs and fears. The behavior of people is often influenced by beliefs and fears they adopt in response to childhood circumstances that are no longer relevant in adulthood. Oftentimes, people are unaware of even having these core beliefs and fears, but still they perpetuate many of the self-defeating behaviors and habits identified in this book. For example, if a person assumes that revealing weaknesses automatically leads to rejection, he or she will conceal vulnerability.

Following are statements of hidden assumptions and fears:

If I merge with you...I will be okay.

The needs of other people...are always more important than my own needs.

It is wrong to say "no"...when others need me. If there is any break in my connection with another...I will be all alone.

If I put you at ease...I am safe.

If I say "no"...I will be rejected.

If I disappoint someone...I am wrong.

I must sacrifice my needs...to preserve harmony.

If I am not "in control"...I will end up like my parents.

My esteem...depends on people liking me.

If I cannot solve your problem...I am a failure.

If I admit weakness...something bad will happen.

If someone is upset...it is my job to take away their discomfort.

I cannot count on others...so I must be self-reliant.

Uncertainty...leads to things getting "out of control."

Can you relate to any of these assumptions?

Ask yourself the following questions :

If I challenge these assumptions, what is the worst thing that could happen?

Are my assumptions an accurate portrayal of my adult life, or are they based on my experiences as a child?

Exercise 5: Discovering/Challenging Assumptions that Squelch Vulnerability

The following questions can be helpful in identifying assumptions that perpetuate "being strong" and "in control."

What would have happened if, as a youngster, you had been LESS responsible in your family? Why is failing wrong?

_____

_____

Do you experience any discomfort when you think about allowing someone to nurture you?

_____

_____

What is your greatest fear regarding letting go of control?

_____

_____

What was it like to express vulnerable emotions in your family?

_____

_____

Recall a situation where you were in a helping role. Imagine that person needing your help, yet none of your efforts can solve their problem(s). What do you feel?

_____

_____

Many people in helping roles define themselves by their ability to give to others and be strong. As a result, they frequently find it difficult to ask others for help, to take their own needs seriously, and to relinquish control. Learning to accept weaknesses, limitations, and powerlessness while learning to feel safe with realistic expectations reduces stress, helps identify realistic limits, and eases the process of reaching out for support.

CHAPTER III

Recreating the Familiar: Childhood Scenarios at Work

The attraction to helping people may be influenced by many factors, some of them not immediately apparent. In a person's attempt to be helpful to others, he or she may perpetuate in adulthood familiar destructive habits and dramas from childhood. For example, people who grow up attending to the needs of family members are often, as adults, drawn to needy people.

What roles did you play growing up in your family?

How did you get attention and/or avoid adverse consequences?

The following questions are designed to help you become aware of how family circumstances may influence one's attraction to a helping role and also perpetuate self-defeating habits.

How Clear Were the Boundaries in Your Family?

Clear boundaries enable people to set limits, maintain a healthy distance, and be compassionate without "taking on" the problems of other people. Ideally, parents attend to their children's needs and do not lean on them for support. Boundaries become blurred when young children and parents are functioning on the same level, such as when children become caretakers or confidantes for their parents.

Frank, the social worker who absorbs people's problems and takes on too much responsibility, grew up being a confidante to his mother. Frank was extremely sensitive to his mother's emotional state and tended to absorb her pain. By confiding her problems to her son, Frank's mother crossed boundaries, using him to meet her own needs.

In addition to absorbing his mother's feelings, Frank learned that his mother's needs and feelings were always more important than his own. Consequently, Frank grew up with a lack of clarity in boundaries that created problems in his adult relationships. He was drawn to people who were needy or in crisis, yet he found it extremely difficult, if not impossible, to ask others for support when he needed it himself.

What were the boundaries like in your family?

_____

_____

_____

Did adults respect your privacy?

_____

_____

_____

Were the adults in your life overprotective, smothering, or domineering?

_____

_____

Were your parents too permissive, perhaps by not setting enough limits or by failing to set clear limits?

_____

_____

_____

How Fair Were the Expectations Placed on You?

Bill is a successful 29-year-old attorney. In the eyes of the world, Bill has everything—good looks, a satisfying career, a supportive girlfriend, and plenty of money. But Bill often feels that he is "not good enough." He continually pushes himself to exhaustion and bases his sense of worth exclusively on his outward achievements.

Bill grew up with a demanding father who expected him to always be the very best at everything he attempted. According to Bill, "Superhuman things were always expected of me. People were depending on me to be a star performer in every area. I could never let Dad down; I had to be good, get all A's in school, be the class president." But no matter how well he performed, Bill never felt like he was good enough.

While Bill's father was overly critical and his excessive expectations were obvious, some parents convey expectations and other messages in unspoken, covert ways. In some families, for example, children may feel pressure to keep the family together by excelling and not making mistakes. No one in the family has to state this expectation, it is simply understood on both sides. Another example of unspoken expectations is evident in a situation where a parent withdraws and gives the "silent treatment" to a child who brings home a report card with all A's and one C. In this case, the unspoken expectation is that one has to be perfect to be valued.

People who grow up with excessive expectations or unrealistic goals thrust upon them are likely to become highly self-critical and perfectionistic as adults. All too often, they are recognized only for their achievements and it appears to them that no one is interested in their "inner person"— their personal thoughts, fears, or concerns. When a person is recognized in this one-dimensional way, a part of that person is denied. The frustration that follows from consistently denying a part of oneself can lead to substance abuse, workaholism, and other compulsive behaviors.

As a Child, Were You Expected To "Be good" and Please Others?

Excessive emphasis on "being good" and pleasing others can undermine a person's ability to manage conflict and set limits. When a child grows up "being good," accommodating, and assuming a caretaker role, he or she often has difficulty recognizing and asserting personal needs and may even neglect self-care.

In some families, "being good," pleasing others, and/or assuming the role of peacekeeper can be effective ways to establish emotional security. For example, when a child is not achieving in a family marked by tension and chaos, that child may fear that things will get "out of control." "Being good" can have the effect of de-escalating tension in families where there is a significant amount of unpre-dictability. In families like this, children learn how to avoid punishment or judgment by behaving so as not to draw attention to themselves and by never making waves. Children who grow up in this kind of environment become hypervigilant to their surroundings, carefully molding their behavior to fit the perceived expectations of others. Following are some other examples of how "being good" relates to upbringing.

• Growing up in a family with strict rules about what constitutes good and bad behavior, which often forces people into rigid, inflexible thinking.

• Becoming a model child in an attempt to overcompensate for a parent's weaknesses, which may be embarrassing.

• Being good in an attempt to get validation and attention. Some children are rewarded for excelling, for being obedient and compliant, and for putting everyone else's needs before their own. A child may learn that he or she can feel special by being Dad's little helper or by listening to Mom's problems. In some families, this altruism brings parental approval, reinforcing the child's over-identification with "being good."

• Pleasing others and working hard to somehow "fit in" can become an extremely important priority in the life of a child who has been treated like an outsider and/or teased by others. When children are teased or rejected, they may become overly concerned about conforming and not appearing blatantly different. Some children will do anything to avoid being an outsider because their self-esteem is exclusively based on how others perceive them and respond to them.

• Being selfless and "going above and beyond" in helping others may, for some children, be reinforced by religious authorities. A 45-year-old counselor told me this: "I remember being an altar boy—the smell of the incense, the wax dripping off the candles—and feeling so special. The priest would tell me to always remember St. Francis and to never break the rules. I learned that God loved those who were selfless, and that I was supposed to 'give until it hurt.'"

As a youngster, was it necessary for you to please people, to be attentive, or to excel?

---

*Were there consequences if you did **not** behave in this manner?*

Did You Grow Up with Too Much Responsibility?

Many people who are drawn to helping others as adults spent their early years being in helper roles. In fact, they may have taken on many adult responsibilities, including the care of family members. When parents are preoccupied or overwhelmed with their own responsibilities and unable to adequately provide security and comfort, their children grow up being overly self-reliant. Because they essentially raise themselves, these children may miss out on childhood; throughout their lives, these people may find it very difficult to rely on others or ask for help.

Children develop an exaggerated sense of responsibility when the adults in their lives are fragile, needy, self-absorbed, or unpredictable. They brace against feelings of powerlessness by taking on the responsibility of maintaining stability for themselves and the family.

Did you assume a helping role with siblings?

_____

_____

Are you more comfortable being in a "giver" role?

_____

_____

Is your self-worth and identity based on being strong, responsible, and productive?

_____

_____

Is fixing people's problems and handling crises for others a familiar role for you?

_____

_____

Do you frequently feel obligated to others?

_____

_____

As a Child, Were You Discouraged from Acknowledging or Expressing Emotional Needs?

The ways your parents responded to your emotional needs affect how you ultimately care for yourself as an adult. *As a child, was it acceptable for you to show sadness or hurt? To*

*what degree did you feel nurtured, reassured, listened to,
and respected by the adults in your life?*

People who grow up in families in which their
emotional needs are not taken seriously are likely to have
difficulty recognizing their needs and nurturing themselves
as adults.

The emotional needs of a child include: respect,
affection, consistency, and predictability. In families where
the needs of the parents dominate and/or the parents are
self-absorbed or needy, the child's emotional needs may be
responded to in a random and arbitrary fashion. When the
needs of one member of a family dominate, perhaps
because of illness, there may be little energy going toward
the children who are well.

During childhood, some people receive messages from
society, parents, or other significant adults that teach them
to downplay or completely ignore their own needs. These
messages are conveyed either directly or indirectly. Indirect
or unspoken messages are more difficult to detect— both in
the present and in retrospect—but they are every bit as
powerful and memorable as direct and spoken messages.

An example of a message communicated directly is the
following: "You think you're the center of the universe."
The same message can be conveyed indirectly, as it was in
the case of Mark, the police dispatcher. As Mark was
learning to be more vulnerable, he spoke of the indirect
messages he received from his parents: "My dad seemed to
withdraw and disapprove whenever I was displaying
vulnerable feelings. And I remember a particular incident
with my mother that really affected me. At the age of nine,
I fell in the school auditorium and chipped my tooth. My
schoolmates laughed and I ran home in tears. Instead of

comforting me, my mother told me not to take myself so seriously, because no one else did."

Although it may not have been her intention to do so, Mark's mother invalidated her son's feelings in that instance, and in many others as well. This is but one example of the powerful messages that Mark received at an early age: that he could not count on people; that expressing disappointment or requesting comfort is wrong; and that he should not take himself so seriously because other people didn't take him seriously. Mark's upbringing subsequently had a negative impact on his adult life. He continued to ignore his feelings and emotional needs until he was able to change the fixed messages that kept playing through his mind.

Did you receive messages as a child that interfered with your ability to recognize and respond to your emotional needs? What were they?

_____

_____

_____

Are you accustomed to downplaying many of your own needs and/or do you tend to regard everyone else's needs as more important than your own? Give an example.

_____

_____

_____

Do you have difficulty recognizing your needs and limitations? Give an example.

_____

_____

_____

Do you have difficulty focusing on goals? Give an example.

_____

_____

_____

Do you have difficulty trusting others and relying on them?

_____

_____

_____

Exercise 6: Changing Fixed Messages

Subconsciously, we tend to repeat to ourselves the same messages that were communicated to us as children—unless we work diligently to change them. In order to change destructive messages, we must give ourselves conscious self-affirmations on a regular basis.

Think of three messages you tell yourself that undermine your ability to respond to or identify your emotional needs.

Then, write the opposite messages and say them aloud.

Examples:

Familiar Message	Opposite Message
1. "I have no right to complain."	"There are circumstances when I have a perfect right to complain."
2. "People will be angry with me if I express sadness."	"It is okay for me to express sadness, and I don't require the approval of others in doing so."
3. "I cannot count on anyone."	"There are people in my life I can count on."
4. "My needs are a burden on others."	"My needs are not necessarily a burden on others and I can express them."

Now, list some of your own negative messages and the corresponding affirmations here:

Familiar Message	Opposite Message

5. _____

_____

_____

6. _____

_____

_____

7. _____

_____

_____

Cultural Considerations

Our attitudes and behaviors are shaped by societal expectations as well as family dynamics. For example, many men are taught that it is wrong to be vulnerable, while women are encouraged to be nurturers. Some cultures emphasize pleasing others, compliance, and non-assertion. Are there cultural factors that influence your helping style?

Consider the circumstances and scenarios in your own family and in your own childhood that you may be recreating in your adult life—both personally and professionally. Identifying the familiar and how it works or doesn't work for you now can break the cycle of self-defeating habits and enhance your capacity to care for yourself.

CHAPTER IV
Saying "Yes" to Yourself

Throughout this book, I have described how people in helping roles often play out familiar scenarios from their upbringing that undermine their effectiveness and cause them to neglect their own needs.

Actually, some people in helping roles regard any focus on themselves as a selfish distraction. But attending to one's own needs and care is not selfishness at all, it is enlightened self-interest. The selfish person seeks instant gratification and is preoccupied with himself or herself to the point of being insensitive to the needs of the others. Enlightened self-interest, however, is acting in accordance with one's own best interests, while being sensitive to the needs of others.

Following is a simple example of enlightened self-interest: Bob had advance dinner plans with Jim for Friday evening. On Wednesday morning, Bob sensed that his energy was beginning to drop. He'd had a busy and exhausting week; by Wednesday evening, he realized that he'd need some time alone at the end of the week. Bob's capacity to detect his own need and respond to it resulted in rescheduling his dinner plans with Jim in a timely way.

Self-Neglect

A key component in self-care is self-awareness. It is important to identify both subtle and obvious ways people in helping roles neglect themselves, as well as the underlying attitudes that perpetuate self-neglect.

Following are common forms of self-neglect:

- Procrastinating — particularly in setting and pursuing goals.

- Failing to take breaks at work.

- "Settling" for difficult working conditions for prolonged periods of time.

- Tolerating insensitive treatment from others.

- Not expressing wants or needs, unless or until the situation is urgent.

- Continually being "on the edge" financially.

Although social conditions contribute to these behaviors, poor self-esteem often fuels self-neglect. For some, deprivation may become a familiar way of life. People who grow up having their feelings negated and/or being rewarded for making everyone else's needs more important than their own frequently assume that they do not deserve happiness or success.

The overworked caregivers must learn to put themselves first in order to strengthen their own self-esteem. Even though it may feel uncomfortable at first, persons who care for others need to look beyond the social conditions that they believe may be causing all of their stress, and focus on what they may be doing to deprive themselves of wholeness and health. Once they begin to meet their own needs by taking care of themselves first, they may find that they have more energy for others. In addition, with each successful action on their own behalf, they will gain the insight and strength necessary to let go of their dependence on others for their good feelings.

Exercise 7: Self-Care Inventory

You may take good care of yourself in some ways, yet neglect yourself in others. For example, you may be attuned to your financial security, but remain socially isolated. The following statements are designed to help you identify areas of your life that you may be neglecting. Next to each item, circle the number that best describes you in the past three months:

	I take excellent care of myself				I take poor care of myself
I regularly engage in activities that nourish me.	5	4	3	2	1
I have supportive friends whom I see regularly.	5	4	3	2	1
I allow others to give to me.	5	4	3	2	1
I can ask others for help.	5	4	3	2	1
I take care of my body— I exercise regularly and have a healthy diet.	5	4	3	2	1
I feel that I deserve to have loving relationships and financial security.	5	4	3	2	1
I make time for leisure, regarding it as a priority.	5	4	3	2	1
I generally know and express how I want to be treated by others.	5	4	3	2	1
I avoid relationships that are not good for me.	5	4	3	2	1
I treat myself with compassion and am tolerant when I make mistakes.	5	4	3	2	1

Getting Needs Met Directly

Emotional-based needs include: human connection, respect, acceptance, and understanding. Because emotional-based needs are more difficult to detect than physical needs, people often attempt to get these needs met in indirect ways. Some of these needs may exist on a subconscious level only, but they are just as powerful in the ways they influence behavior. For example, when people feel lonely or need human contact, they may not be conscious of their needs. They are aware, however, that they feel uncomfortable. But instead of contacting a friend for support, they may may eat, drink, gamble, or shop in order to feel comfortable and nurtured.

Focusing on Yourself

People in helping roles spend a great deal of time and energy being focused on others. This over-involvement with others may actually be a way of avoiding uncomfortable emotions or an attempt to insure acceptance by others. In fact, people learn to detach from their feelings, which also may prevent them from identifying their needs. They may have difficulty recognizing the emotions and/or physical sensations that might serve to alert other people to the fact that they're becoming overextended.

People learn to deepen their contact with themselves by "listening" to the inner workings of their own bodies. Meditation teacher Suzuki Roshi writes about cultivating a listening mind. He suggests learning first to quiet the mind and suspend opinions, judgments, and the tendency to "figure things out" analytically. It is through sensing in this way that we become attuned to subtle cues, such as a queasiness in the stomach or shallow breathing.

When we are attuned to—and take seriously—our sensations, feelings, perceptions and intuitions, we are guided toward personal direction and are able to identify both general and specific needs. For example, a general need is the desire for more supportive friendships; a specific need is preferring support from a friend at a given moment.

Not only is it important for people in helping roles to cultivate better self-awareness, but they also need to address beliefs that interfere with their capacity to focus on themselves. In addition to having a fear of rejection and an "addiction to harmony," many people in helping roles view their own needs as relatively unimportant. They need to examine these issues, think about their "preferences," and how they wish to be treated by others. It may be useful for them to ask themselves whether their helper roles as children resulted in being recognized and valued by the family. They also need to learn to "listen" to themselves.

Recharging Your Battery

Many people involved in helping others have much more energy going out to others than they have energy coming back to them. Indeed, they are accustomed to making everyone else's needs more important than their own needs, which prevents them from tending to important aspects of self-care: setting limits, pursuing their own interests and goals, and saying "no" to those who treat them in an insensitive manner. People in helping roles need to learn healthy ways to take care of themselves. By doing so, they will be helping others in healthier ways. Learning to take care of oneself involves, among other things, paying attention to personal health matters, actively seeking supportive relationships, and making time for leisure activities.

Exercise 8: Direct Communication

Many people have difficulty identifying emotional-based needs, particularly if they have never learned how to ask for what they want or if they feel that they have "no right" to make requests of others. Expression of needs requires being vulnerable and direct, and it's often easier to resort to blame or withdrawal. Asking for what you want and revealing your emotional needs does not guarantee that those needs automatically will be met. Being direct, however, can increase the likelihood of getting want you need.

Think of someone who is important in your life; then think back to a situation when you would have liked that person to respond differently to you. (It is important to choose someone who is capable of hearing your requests without negating you.) Describe the situation.

_____

_____

What are you needing emotionally? Be specific!

_____

_____

Now imagine that this person is in front of you at this moment. Tell him or her what you need, beginning with this clear statement: "What I need from you is…"

_____

_____

After you make your statement to this person, notice how you felt doing this exercise and write about it here.

My Reaction:

_____

_____

Your Support Network: Who Takes Care of You While You're Taking Care of Others?

It bears repeating: many people in helping roles are much better at attending to the needs of others than they are at caring for themselves. To add to the problem, they frequently have difficulty asking for help, which increases the likelihood of burnout. Helpers who work in a private practice setting are often isolated from other professionals. Working in an agency, hospital, or organization also can create a unique sense of isolation. One useful practice is budgeting time during work meetings to discuss personal concerns related to work. Another helpful idea is to cultivate friendships with people who do not expect you to be "strong."

Exercise 9: Establishing a Committed Relationship with Yourself

Imagine...you are upset and choose to confide in someone who is very concerned about you...

Notice the way this concerned person listens to you—the tone of voice and his/her body language.

Now, when this image becomes clear, imagine that the person you are envisioning is you...responding to you in this same comforting manner.

What was your reaction when you imagined your response toward yourself?

_____

_____

_____

Frank, the social worker who absorbed the problems of his clients, is an example of a helping person who learned to form a committed relationship with himself. For the first time in his life, Frank began to pay attention to what he wanted, and also began spending time just for himself. He became involved in several activities that reflected his personal interests: hobbies, visiting friends, and going to the gym.

Frank also set aside specific blocks of time each week for his preferred activities, making specific appointments "with himself" in his weekly calendar. Previously, any thoughts or plans like this would have resulted in his judging his activities as selfish. Frank's former behavior was guided by his perception of how others would respond to him rather than by his own instincts and interests.

People in helping roles often need reminders to take care of themselves since it is so easy for them to forget that they are susceptible to falling back into the pattern of unhealthy caretaking. Activities that can tangibly engage the caregivers in an ongoing personal inventory of behaviors and beliefs may successfully keep them consciously involved in taking care of their own needs.

In addition to the exercises presented thus far in this booklet, this chapter contains exercises to help caretakers identify and work with areas of their lives which can be problematic. The exercises help to increase awareness and to remind caregivers of their commitment to self-care. This increased awareness and commitment can accomplish much in changing destructive and unhealthy patterns of self-neglect that contribute so heavily to burnout among persons who devote the majority of their time to helping others.

The Self-Care Inventory on page 47 can also be used as a periodic check-up to keep track of how you, as a caregiver, are taking good care of yourself as well as others. It can serve as a continuing reminder that your needs are important and that you, too, deserve good treatment.

The Self-Care Wheel is a particularly useful tool, also. Use it to remind yourself of the areas in which you can focus for enlightened self-interest, rather than selfishness.

Self-Care Wheel: How Are You Doing?

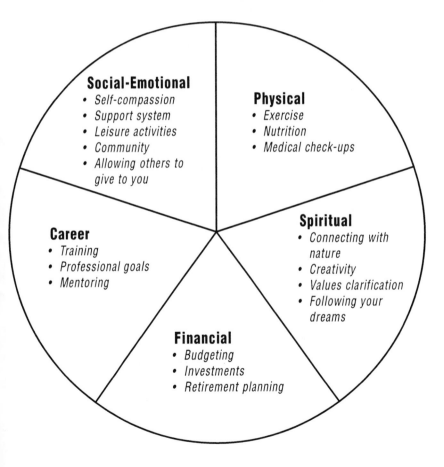

Social-Emotional
- Self-compassion
- Support system
- Leisure activities
- Community
- Allowing others to give to you

Physical
- Exercise
- Nutrition
- Medical check-ups

Career
- Training
- Professional goals
- Mentoring

Spiritual
- Connecting with nature
- Creativity
- Values clarification
- Following your dreams

Financial
- Budgeting
- Investments
- Retirement planning

It may be helpful to refer to the Self-Care Wheel periodically to assist you in maintaining a healthy balance in your life. By conscientiously monitoring your self-care practices, you can stay focused and protect yourself against stress, self-neglect, and burnout.

Additional Strategies for Improving and Maintaining the Quality of Self-Care

Take Breaks. Many people in helping roles forget to take breaks while at work. In some situations, if they do take a break, they feel guilty or sense—sometimes accurately, sometimes not—resentment from coworkers. It is helpful to discuss breaks in work meetings in order to cultivate a climate of mutual support.

Exercise. Demanding or troubled clients and customers can remain in your thoughts and feelings when you are away from work. Exercise is a good way of "cleaning out" the events and tasks related to these work-related stresses. Of course, exercise also builds resilience to stress and offers balance to people whose work requires an emphasis on mental activity.

Maintain a life outside of your helping role. Many caregivers spend too much of their time and energy attending to others. Make time for solitude as well as for personal and professional enrichments, hobbies, and nurturing relationships.

Make a list of healthy things you do to nurture yourself. Set aside some time each week to do the activities you would like to do and consciously schedule time for leisure. Treat that designated leisure time with the same priority you would any important meeting.

Strive to achieve and sustain a healthy balance. Some people grow up in families where having fun is acceptable only after all the work is done. Most people in helping roles find that their work is never really done. The ongoing challenge of helping others, for all its rewards, calls for ongoing efforts related to self-care.

Consider the following simple adjustments to create positive change in your life.

Hire someone to clean the house.

Take the allotted breaks at work.

Take time for quiet and solitude.

Spend more time with friends and other people who are caring and nurturing.

Meditate.

Sign up for—and attend—classes of your own choosing.

Spend time enjoying nature.

Exercise regularly.

Get a massage on a regular basis.

Design a self-care plan. Think about what you can do to take better care of yourself, including all that you have learned about yourself and what you need to do to accomplish that. Don't forget to include the tools you have been given here in this chapter. Exercise 10 gives you a format to use in designing your plan.

Exercise 10: My Self-Care Plan

Based on your review of the self-care evaluation in this section, write a paragraph below outlining some new ways you can improve the quality of your self-care:

_____

_____

_____

_____

_____

_____

_____

_____

_____

_____

_____

_____

Self-Care Weekly Calendar

It is important for people in helping roles to periodically review their self-care, along with their needs and action plans to meet those needs. Set aside specific times each week to participate in activities that are pleasing and/or restful for you.

Make it a point to do something nurturing for yourself each and every day. And to insure that these special plans don't get lost in the shuffle, place them on your calendar at the beginning of the month and honor them just as you would any other personal or professional engagement.

Self-Care Weekly Calendar

	Mon	Tues.	Wed.	Thurs.	Fri.	Sat.	Sun.
9 am							
10 am							
11 am							
12 N							
1 pm							
2 pm							
3 pm							
4 pm							
5 pm							
6 pm							
7 pm							
8 pm							
9 pm							

The Self-Care Assessment below is a good tool to use for identifying beliefs that are creating overly responsible behavior on your part, patterns from childhood that still may be driving you in your overidentification as a caretaker of others, and areas in which you are neglecting yourself. By filling it out and studying your score, you may see new information emerging that can help you accept the reality of your situation. Awareness is the first step toward change. And with change, you can free yourself from self-imposed stress, overwork, fatigue, and all the other characteristics described in this book.

After you have completed the assessment, check your plan for self-care and make adjustments if necessary, so that you can start to enjoy the life you have while helping others to enjoy theirs.

Self-Care: An Assessment

Consider the following 40 statements below, filling in the blanks that follow with the number that best corresponds with your life at this time.

Responses: 1= Very True

2= Somewhat True

3= Rarely True

1. When people get upset, I try to smooth things out._____

2. I am able to listen to other people's problems without trying to "fix"them and/or take away their pain._____

3. My self-worth is determined by how others perceive me._____

4. When I am exposed to conflict, I feel it is my fault._____

5. When my actions somehow cause disappointment for others, I feel guilty._____

6. When I make a mistake, I tend to be extremely critical of myself; I have difficulty forgiving myself._____

7. I usually know how I want other people to treat me._____

8. I tell people how I prefer to be treated._____

9. My achievements define my self-worth._____

10. I feel anxious in most situations involving confrontation._____

11. In relationships, it is easier for me to "give" than to "receive."_____

12. I can be so focused on someone I am helping that I lose sight of my own perceptions, interests, and desires._____

13. It is hard for me to express sadness._____

14. To make mistakes means that I am weak._____

15. It is best to not "rock the boat" or "make waves."_____

16. It is important to put people at ease._____

17. It is best not to need others._____

18. If I cannot solve a problem, I feel like a failure._____

19. I often feel "used up" at the end of the day._____

20. I take work home frequently._____

21. I can ask for help only if the situation is serious._____

22. I am willing to sacrifice my needs in order to please others._____

23. When faced with uncertainty, I feel that things will get totally out of control._____

24. I am uncomfortable when others do not see me as being strong and self-sufficient.____

25. In intimate relationships, I am drawn to people who are needy or who need me.____

26. I can express my differing opinion in the face of an opposing viewpoint.____

27. When I say "no," I feel guilty.____

28. When others distance from me, I feel anxious.____

29. When listening to someone's problems, I am more aware of their feelings than I am of my own feelings. ____

30. I stand up for myself and express my feelings when someone treats me in an insensitive manner.____

31. I feel anxious when I am not busy.____

32. I believe that expressing resentments is wrong.____

33. I am more comfortable giving than receiving.____

34. I become anxious when I think I've disappointed someone.____

35. Work dominates much of my life.____

36. I seem to be working harder and accomplishing less.____

37. I feel most worthwhile and alive in crisis situations.____

38. I have difficulty saying "no" and setting limits.____

39. My interests and values reflect what others expect of me rather than my own interests and values.____

40. People rely on me for support.____

It is important for people in helping roles to periodically review their self-care, along with their needs and action plans to meet those needs.

If you find that you've responded with a 1 (Very True) to more than 15 of these items, it's time to take a close and careful look at self-care issues.

◆

SELECTED REFERENCES

"Altruism as Value-Centered Action." In *Noetic Science Review*, 1990.

"Burnout and Health Workers." In *Hospital Magazine*, 1979: Vol 43.

Deutsch C. "Self-reported sources of stress among psychotherapists." In *Professional Psychology Research and Practice*, 1984: Vol 15, p. 833.

Figley, C. *Compassion Fatigue: Coping with Secondary Traumatic Stress*. New York, NY: Brunner/Mazel, 1995.

Larson, D. *The Helper's Journey*. Champaign, Illinois: Research Press, 1993.

Love, P. *The Emotional Incest Syndrome*. New York: Bantam, 1990.

Moore, T. *Care of The Soul*. New York: Harper/Collins, 1994.

"Nurses Who Give Too Much." In *American Journal of Nursing*, 1989: Vol. 11.

Patrick, P. "Professionals at Risk for Burnout." In *Family and Community Health*, 1984: Vol. 6 pp. 25-31.

Perlman and McCann. "Vicarious Trauma." In *Journal of Traumatic Stress*, 1990: Vol. 3 #1.

Portnoy, D. "Are You Caring or Caretaking?" In *Journal of Hospice and Palliative Care*, May 1993.

Suzuki, S. *Zen Mind, Beginner's Mind* New York/Toyko: Weatherhill, 1970.

Snow, C. *I'm Dying to Take Care of You.* Deerfield Beach, Florida: Professional Counselor Books/Health Communications, 1990.

"Take Three Nurses." In *Nursing Times*, December 1991: Vol. 87

Woititz, J. *Home Away From Home.* Deerfield Beach, Florida: Health Communications, 1987.

About the Author

Dennis Portnoy is a licensed counselor in private practice in San Francisco. One of his specializations is assisting people in helping roles to identify and counteract the self-defeating aspects of unhealthy helping. Mr. Portnoy's message is that familiar childhood roles, personality traits, and beliefs hold the key to improving effectiveness and minimizing the negative effects of stress. Recognizing that people in helping roles are particularly vulnerable in today's volatile and demanding work climate, he devotes much of his time to lecturing, training, and teaching people to prevent burnout and to take care of themselves in healthy ways while taking care of others.

For information about trainings, in-services, seminars, or lectures, write:

1537 Franklin St. #310
San Francisco, CA. 94109

Notes